THE YOUNG LIVING VITALITY FOOD PAIRING BIBLE

INTRODUCTION

In the last few years, it's' no secret essential oils have become quite the craze. Whether you've seen them on the shelves of convenience stores or infused in your favorite shower gels and skin care products, these oils are everywhere. While most people's knowledge of essential oils doesn't extend beyond the idea of their aromas smelling incredibly pleasant drifting throughout our homes, my experience with the Young Living Vitality oils has taught me that there are so many other ways to use them. Essential oils aren't just for aromatherapy and diffusers anymore, certain oils (provided they are pure, all natural, and of high quality) can be incredibly powerful tools useful in the kitchen. This may seem far-fetched at first, but when you think about it, essential oils are simply concentrated derivatives of the natural oils found in plants we consume on a regular basis, just in whole form. When properly distilled they are safe to use topically and through ingestion (as in diffusing, taking orally, or infused in foods and beverages). To make this concept totally clear, essential oils are very similar to extracts you already keep in your kitchen, like vanilla or lemon, but they're way more potent and all natural.

Before moving forward, it's crucial that I mention that not all essential oils are created equal. Despite their supply being widely available and often sold by stores we trust, many oils in the marketplace are for aromatherapy and/or topical use and are not suitable for human consumption. Before experimenting with ingesting oils or adding them to your favorite recipe, make sure they're approved for ingestion or considered food grade. Young Living Vitality oils are one of the only FDA approved brands approved for ingestion and subsequently, the focus of the following text. Their Seed to Seal® program is their quality standard. The three pillars of this meticulous approach—Sourcing, Science, and Standards—allow them to deliver pure, authentic essential oils and essential oil-infused products that you and your family can use with full peace of mind.

Although the recent surge in people using essential oils more domestically has increased, few people have transitioned to using them in the kitchen on a regular basis outside of recipes they've stumbled upon here and there. It's plausible to think this is due to people's natural tendency to be skeptical about using the oils in an unfamiliar way, or simply because they just haven't thought about it yet. Either way, past precedent alone suggests cooking with essential oils is nothing new, especially considering their wide use commercially. Although the food industry primarily uses essential oils as flavoring agents, it's worth mentioning they represent an interesting source of natural antimicrobials useful for food preservation.

It's important to note that when using essential oils as food preservatives, it's imperative to establish detailed knowledge about the oils scientific properties, the ratios required to emit the oils anti-spoilage capabilities, and express knowledge of the oils effects on the foods intended for preservation. With that being said, the scope of the coming text is largely focused on essentials oil's ability to accent and flavor foods. Truthfully, most of us consume essential oils regularly, we often just don't know it. Some examples of foods infused with essential oils range from puddings, chewing gums, sauces, salad dressings, herbal teas, ice creams, popsicles and more: Even "all natural" toothpaste is flavored with essential oils.

The information you'll learn in the coming pages is intended to spark your creative juices so that you may continue enjoying the benefits of essential oils in yet another powerful way. Although, we won't get into specific recipes the descriptions of the Young Living Vitality oils serves as the foundation for you to begin building incredible dishes. We often refer to cooking as culinary art, and as with all art, every great masterpiece begins with a vision. Our vision with cooking involves thoughtful combination and manipulation of various ingredients. Amazing cooking involves balancing those flavors harmoniously. I once heard that the trait of a great meal is when the flavors of a dish are vibrant, but simultaneously undetectable. Undoubtedly, by developing an understanding of each of the oils distinct characteristics and how their flavor profiles pair with other foods, you'll begin to envision cheful master pieces of your own. No matter what your skill level is in the kitchen, learning to improve the overall flavor of your food is within the realm of possibility for everyone, especially with the ease of using essential oils.

COOKING WITH ESSENTIAL OILS

As you begin experimenting in the kitchen, I encourage you to remember these three principles that will guide your journey and improve your rate of success while cooking with essential oils.

Conversion

Essential oils are concentrated derivatives of their original sources meaning they're very powerful and packed with flavor. As a rule of thumb, when using oils in the kitchen, a little goes a long way. Start with simply 1 drop at a time and for the most part, try to avoid adding essential oils directly into your dishes unless you're baking or making a large batch of something like a soup or stew. Even in these scenarios, a fraction of a drop may be sufficient for the entire recipe depending on the herb or spice you're using. Unfortunately, there is no exact science to converting oils or applying ratios to recipes; what works in one scenario may not apply to another. For instance, the flavor in citrus oil tends to be less intense compared to traditional culinary herbs like basil or dill oil. For this reason, your approach to using them in recipes is going to be very different. So when trying to figure out how much essential oil is needed in a recipe ask yourself a question: What is my intention in using this particular oil? If your intention is to make the essential oil be the star of the dish, obviously you'll need to add more than you would if your only seeking to add subtle notes of that particular flavor in your dish, and vice versa.

Fusion

Fusion is one of the most practical methods for using essential oils in the kitchen. It's also a great way to stretch the dollars you spend on them. One of the great things about this approach is that it's not complicated; in fact it's rather easy. To begin creating your own infusions, you simply add your favorite essential oils directly into lipids. From a culinary perspective lipids are simply a fats and there are plenty of healthy fats to begin experimenting with. The purpose of adding essential oils to lipids is multifaceted. First, it helps to reduce the intensity of the oils over arching flavor. Additionally, it allows the flavor of the herb or spice to spread evenly throughout the dish. The best part about creating your own infusions with essential oils is they generally never go rancid, so you're able to use them until they're finished. Below are a few formulas to help guide your experimentation with fusion. I've also created a list of acceptable lipids that lend well to creating your own infusions. As mentioned earlier, try to avoid adding essential oils directly into your recipes unless your adding them directly to baked goods, stocks, stews, soups, naturally fatty dishes like guacamole or cream sauces.

Formula for Infusing Lipids

1 cup lipid + 3-5 drops (depending on the intensity) essential oil = Infused oil

Formula to split 1 drop of Oil

1 drop + 1 teaspoon of lipid (use a calibrated medicine spoon)
(from here you can use ⅛ tsp, ¼ tsp, ½ tsp etc.)

Lipids

Almond oil	Coconut oil	Sesame oil
Avocado oil	Corn oil	Sunflower oil
Mustard oil	Flaxseed oil	Grape seed oil
Butter	Olive oil	Vegetable oil blend
Butter Clarified	Palm oil	
Canola oil	Peanut oil	

Timing

As with most herbs and spices, the timing in which you add them to your recipe can play an extremely critical role in the outcome of your overall dish. Naturally, as with their whole counterparts, it's better to add some oils in at the beginning of the recipe and others towards the end of the cooking process. Contrary to many misconceptions, a lengthy cooking process or heat in general does not diminish the flavor of essential oils. It can actually have a balancing effect on some essential oils raw harshness. On the flip side, heat neutralizes essential oils health-supporting qualities. So keep this in mind when preparing recipes that require heat to allow for proper cooling before adding essential oils if your intention is to benefit from their wellness promoting properties.

*Citrus oils are commonly used in natural food preservation; however, their antimicrobial properties are ineffective if added to hot food.

ESSENTIAL OILS AND YOUR PALATE

Great food isn't simply the product of following a specific recipe; if it were, everyone would be a great cook, right? Great food only happens when the preparer has intentionally balanced the flavors. This can only happen when a person has developed their palate and, sadly, it's rarely taught. Many of us use the terms "flavor" and "taste" interchangeably, but modern science defines these terms as two totally separate things. The entire process is very intimate when you think about it because nobody experiences flavor and taste in the same way. This is due to every flavor impression being based on stimulus from three senses: taste, smell, and touch, the latter being the smell of food exhaled through the nose during chewing or after swallowing. Breathing is a natural occurrence, so even while chewing and swallowing you always exhale air through your nose. This air passes the olfactory tissue in the back of the nose which manifest the experience of flavor. It's estimated that about 85% of what we perceive of as flavor is really impressions processed in our nasal system. It's the sense of smell, or lack thereof, that makes it difficult to enjoy food when you're feeling under the weather. When your sick and congested you're unable to smell food in the same capacity as when you're well. As a result, your sense of flavor is only limited to the information processed by your palate.

Taste, unlike flavor, is interpreted more dominantly in the palate and thought to be broken into five categories: sweet, sour, salty, bitter, and umami (which is considered a rich savory impression). Our ability to sense these five accepted categories comes from receptors on our taste buds and throughout our palates. These tiny sensory organs appear mostly on the tongue, the roof of our mouth, and in the back of the throat.

In addition to our taste buds and olfactory system working together, there are two other components that play a role in our capacity to experience flavor. These are our sense of touch and our mind's ability to remember the aromas and flavors we perceive. Cooking, at it's heart, is the creative act of transforming food through various means of temperature and machinery. The ability to manipulate textures in the cooking process makes it possible for us to experience the same foods in all its various forms. Touch undoubtedly plays a role in how we perceive and interpret foods and beverages. It's because of touch that strong differences of opinion exist over random topics like what's better between pulpy versus smooth orange juice. On a deeper level, our palate's touch sensitivity gives our mouths the ability to sift pin sized fish bones through protein, and detect foreign pieces of plastic before swallowing. It protects us from the moment food hits our mouth to the time we swallow, it even triggers our gag reflex when all else fails to stop us from swallowing foods our bodies deem to be harmful.

The final component in our perception of flavor is our mind, which is the intrinsic force driving our ability to truly enjoy our meals. Our ability to imagine and create memories around food create a narrative for the way we consume, prepare, and interact with food all together. Our memories allow us to keep special moments and people alive through the stories we tell at the dinner table. It's those familiar flavors and smells that we often associate with home, wherever that may be. Below is a breakdown of how the mouth perceives taste sensations as it relates to essential oils.

Five Taste Sensations

Sweet

Sweetness, generally regarded as a pleasurable sensation, is the most fundamental of taste pleasures, it signals the presence of sugars, the foundation of the food chain and a source of energy. The front of your palate is where sweetness is detected. The next time you enjoy a pastry or piece of chocolate, see if you can feel the sensation that occurs at the front of your mouth. Essential oils typically contain trace amounts of sugars, so they'll never present as overly sweet. However, by developing the awareness of where the intensity is most dominant in your mouth, it helps detect sweetness even when there are minimal amounts. A designation of sweet when describing certain oils later in the book will be for oils that lend well to sweet dishes.

Sour

Acids in citrus fruits, vinegars, and other foods cause the mouth-crinkling sensation described as sour. Modern scientist are still debating the biological purpose of this sensation, but many suspect that sourness originally signaled food was decomposing and potentially unsafe to eat. We experience this sour sensation most dominantly on the sides of our tongues, right in the middle on each sides. Most people would suspect citrus oils to emit the sour sensation, however, Young Living citrus oils are cold-pressed right from the skin of the fruit, so the oils are acid free. A designation of sour when describing certain oils later in the book will be for oils that lend well to sour dishes because none of the oils alone embody a sour designation.

Salty

We're hardwired with an inherent sensitivity to salt, which is why the difference between a pinch and a teaspoon can be the difference between a great dish and the worst thing you've ever eaten in your life. Our internal sodium meters help to ensure we consume just the right amount to maintain the healthy balance our bodies need to function optimally. It's common knowledge; overuse of salt throws our bodies out of alignment resulting in sickness and disease. The good news: If you cut back on salt, your taste buds can adapt to be satisfied with less. Saltiness can also be perceived at the front palate, but this sensation stretches a little farther to the sides of your front palate.

Bitter

Bitterness is a distinctive bad taste accompanied by an equally disgusted facial expression that screams to the world "I just ate something gross". A variety of substances, mostly found in plants, emanate a noticeably bitter element, which is the case for most of our essential oils. Although bitterness isn't pleasant to experience on it's own, when accompanied with other ingredients, a touch of bitterness in food becomes interesting, yet equally balanced. The middle to back region of the tongue is where you sense bitterness. If you're unsure of what this sensation is like, try a piece of arugula or extremely dark chocolate. A designation of bitter when describing essential oils pertains to the flavor of the oil and not the dish.

Umami

Umami roughly translates to "delicious" in Japanese. It's kind of hard to describe, it's not quite sweet, it's not really salty, it's just one of those sensations that embodies the concept of full-flavored. That deep, rich, primal intensity that distinguishes a fried egg from a boiled egg. It's that flavor savoring essence of soy sauce, mushrooms, smoked Gouda, and bacon, among other things. In the simplest terms, umami actually comes from glutamates and a group of chemicals called ribonucleotides, which also occur naturally in many foods. When you combine ingredients containing these different umami-giving properties, they enhance one another to create flavors that are out of this world. Even the most primitive of foods like potatoes and ketchup pack massive umami kick with minimal effort by the preparer. Incredible results can be obtained by simply combining ingredients in umami-enhancing ways. Umami it hits the back of your throat and leaves you craving more. Essential oils that carry this designation will leave flavors on your palate lingering long after the meal is finished.

Consider a person with a sophisticated palate, something that can be acquired (no one's born with one); you'd imagine they've developed a keen sense of the five taste sensations. You'd probably also suspect their interest in connecting and experiencing food wouldn't stop there. A classic aficionado wouldn't limit themselves to only 5 descriptive terms for distinguishing their affinity for food, especially when describing herbs and spices, which are seemingly the flavor building blocks of a dish. The taste sensations are incredibly useful tools for understanding how we perceive flavor, but alone, they're not quite expressive enough to convey the true flavor profiles of essential oils. In my opinion, they apply more broadly to completed dishes or stand alone foods that can be consumed on their own, like a lemon (sour) or peach (sweet).

When you consider the strong aromatic properties of herbs and spices there are several more flavor classifications that come to mind for describing them, this is especially useful because most of them have more than one flavor profile in the first place. For example, the commonly used spice cinnamon falls into a few descriptive categories, as it is both woodsy and spicy. For the case of essential oils cinnamon even exhibits a mild floral element. Rosemary is pungent, savory, herbaceous, and piney. By becoming more aware of what we experience on our palates, we simultaneously train our minds to recognize the many flavors, aromas, and tactile sensations this beautiful world has to offer. Below you will find some commonly used sensory characteristics when describing the flavors and aroma profiles of essential oils.

Additional Sensory Impressions

Cooling

Cooling oils exhibit a refreshing sensation. You experience the curiously strong cold flavor when eating a chocolate mint or after rinsing with mouthwash.

Earthy

Earthy spices are those which possess a rustic, mineral-like flavor. These are associated with root vegetables, seeds, and other varieties growing underground or in the deep forest. It almost like the taste closely resembles where they where grown.

Floral

Floral spices possess a pleasant aroma similar to the smell of fresh flowers on a summer day. You can often find this flavors reflected in herbal teas and refreshing beverages.

Citrusy

Although it's not quite specific, spices with this designation exhibit a semi-sweet, fruit-like undertone. The fruit flavor can range from a singular expression-as in a lemony zing-or an amalgamation of flavors-such as citrus punch.

Herbaceous

Herbaceous flavors are the ones that taste like you would think "plants" taste like in their rawest form. I'm not talking about plants with fruit either, think of green leaves and sprouts, when trying to conceptualize this flavor.

Nutty

This flavor taste exactly how it sounds. In the most basic form of nuts, I tend to think of peanuts, but call to mind whatever nuts works for you to create the impression. There is almost something buttery about the nutty flavor.

Piney

When I think of piney, I tend to think of Christmas. If you have ever smelled a Christmas tree before, you have a vague sense of what the pine flavor tastes like. The aromatic scent of piney properties are so strong they accompany a mildly minty flavor in the back of your palate when inhales closely. It's distinct smell with a pleasant bite that one can easily learn to love.

Pungent

Spices that fall under the pungent classification are extreme in flavor and have strong aromatics as well. They typically don't play well with other spices, so be sure to dilute them before adding them to your dish.

Spicy

Oils that are classified as spicy give a powerful burst of flavor and heat simultaneously. What separates spicy from hot is that spicy sensations, although intense, are short lived where hot just continues.

Woodsy

When I think of woodsy, I think of the actual woods. These are the flavors that taste vaguely like the food has been smoked over a wooden-burning stove. It's like the cedar flavor is absorbed when cooking on a cedar plank or the smokiness of a wild mushroom when added to a recipe.

ESSENTIAL OIL TEMPERATURES

You may have heard essential oils referred to as "hot" but were not sure exactly what that meant. The reality is, it's exactly what you'd expect it to mean especially when using Young Living essential oils. When dealing with high quality therapeutic oils they can be dangerous if mishandled or abused. Warm and hot oils have properties that exhibit heat when applied to the skin or ingested. "Hot" in a sense of taste is characterized by its ability to heat up your mouth quickly, sometimes making food unpleasant or in some cases undesirable all together.

One important consideration to remember is that everyone experiences oils in their own unique interpretation. So what may be warm or hot to one person, may not be as intense for others, however, some oils are just hot, like oregano, and should be handled with care. For scenarios like this it's always recommended to dilute using a carrier oil. If you experience a "hot" sensation when using an oil, flush the area thoroughly with a carrier oil, such as a high quality, cold-pressed olive oil — this includes your eye. You do not want to flush with water as this may spread the oil to other areas causing a greater depth of that intense "hot" sensation. Flush only with a carrier oil as the fat of the oil will draw the essential oil to it.

Intensity

An incredibly significant consideration when cooking with essential oils is the oils "intensity". As mentioned throughout the text Vitality oils are extremely potent products, but even within this extreme group of flavors, their intensity is displayed over a spectrum. To help make sense of this, think of exercising on treadmill with an incline and speed of "1" indicating a "mild" oil like lemon, and the difference in intensity between an incline and speed of "10" signaling a "severe" oil like rosemary. Naturally, to balance your dish you'll need to use them differently to render contrasting outcomes. The moral to the story is to be aware of an oils intensity when adding it to a recipe, if miscalculated the results can be disastrous.

Purpose

Herbs and spices bring food to life and tell specific stories about the people who've prepared them. Ideally, a potato is a potato, no matter if you're in America or in Europe, but the spices added to it create an entirely different experience when consumed in the different places. The purpose of an herb or spice plays a vital role in how it should be used in a dish. Given all the different properties in plants whole form the most of the same properties transfer to essential oils. While some oils are hot others possess a cooling factor that can greatly enhance a dish. Saltiness tends to stimulate thirst, while sourness counters these effects. Bitterness balances sweetness and adds complexity to a dish, while sweetness on its own evokes feelings of contentment. This is why dessert is usually severed at the end of the meal. Keeping an oils purpose in mind will help you use them more wisely and get the results you're intending.

FOOD PAIRINGS FOR ESSENTIAL OILS

Within the page descriptions of the Vitality oils are flavor profiles for each, as well as food pairings that partner well with each of their unique characteristics. Despite not going into specific recipes, these profiles are thorough reviews of the essential oils usability in the kitchen.

These explanations and examples will hopefully inspire you and broaden your understanding of how essential oils can enhance your meals for years to come.

HOW TO GET STARTED WITH YOUNG LIVING ESSENTIAL OILS

1) Go to: https://www.myyl.com/lisalis411#enroll

2) Confirm you're signing up under Lisa Mitchell Member# 12607265, then begin to make your selections.

3) If you're starting with the Premium Starter Kit click the 'Next' tab to continue. If you'd like to view the full catalog before continuing your enrollment; choose the option that says 'Continue enrollment on Young Living' to customize your order.

4) Fill out your personal information

5) Check the 'terms and conditions' box

6) Be sure to take note of your chosen username, password, and PIN

8)Enter your credit card details and select 'Next'

9)Follow any remaining prompts.

Once you've signed up as a wholesale member and purchased your kit, you will be added to the 'Essential Ed' Facebook group comprised of over 4000 members. As a member of this group you will receive a wealth of free on-going education, suggestions, and usage tips for your new oily journey.

CITRUS OILS

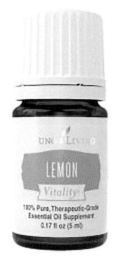

Lemon (Jade Lemon)

Taste: bitter, citrusy

Temperature: hot

Intensity: mild - moderate

Timing: Add at the end of cooking process unless using in baked goods

Purpose: Lemon juice penetrates through the flavors of a dish with an aggressive hit of acidity, lemon oil takes a much more refined approach by gently balancing other flavors while releasing the aroma of freshly-peeled lemons.

Pairs with:

Anise, apples, apricots, anchovies, artichokes, arugula, asparagus, avocado, bananas, barley, basil, bay leaf, black pepper, beef, beer, **Berries**, beans, bean curd, bok choy, broccoli, broccoli rabe, brussel sprouts, buckwheat, butter, buttermilk, capers, caramel, cardamom, cayenne, cauliflower, celery, **Cheese: parmesan, mascarpone**, cherries, chervil, chestnuts, chickpeas, chicken, chili peppers, chives, chocolate, **Citrus fruit**, clams, cinnamon, coconut, coffee, corn, crab, cranberries, cream & **Milk: cow, almond, soy, cashew, coconut**, creme fraiche, cumin, custard, dates, desserts, dill, duck, eggplant, endive, escarole, figs, garlic, ginger, grapefruit, grapes, **Greek cuisine**, green beans, guava, hazelnuts, honey, horseradish, kale, kiwi, kohlrabi, lamb, leeks, lemongrass, lemon verbena, lettuce, lychees, mango, **Mediterranean cuisine**, meringue, mint, **Moroccan cuisine**, mushrooms, mustard, **Nuts**, oats, okra, olives, olive oil, **Onions**, oregano, papaya, paprika, parsley, parsnips, pasta, peaches, pears, persimmons, plums, poppy seeds, pork, poultry, prunes, quince, quinoa, raisins, rhubarb, rosemary, rum, rutabaga, sage, salt, **Sauces**, sesame oil, **Seafood esp. shellfish,** shallots, sherry, snow peas, sour cream, spinach, strawberries, squash, swiss chard, sugar, tequila, thyme, tomatoes, vanilla, vinegar, vodka, walnuts, watercress, **Wine**, yogurt

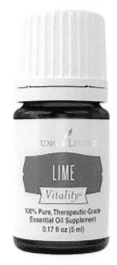

Lime

Taste: bitter

Temperature: citrusy,

Intensity: mild/moderate

Timing: Add at the end of cooking process unless using in baked goods

Purpose: Lime juice, too, is high in acidity, lime oil gently balances flavors while imparting a fierce zing of fresh lime.

Pairs with:

African cuisine (north), Apricots, artichokes, arugula, asparagus, avocados, bananas, basil, black pepper, beef, beer, **Berries**, beans, bean curd, buckwheat, butter, buttermilk, capers, caramel, cayenne, ceviche, cherries, chervil, chestnuts, chickpeas, chicken, chili peppers, chives, chocolate, cilantro, **Citrus fruit**, cinnamon, clams, coconut, coffee, corn, crab, cranberries, cream, creme fraiche, cumin, custard, dates, desserts, duck, figs, garlic, ginger, grapefruit, green tea, guava, hazelnuts, honey, jicama, kiwi, **Latin American cuisine,** lemon, lemongrass, lemon verbena, mangoes, meats esp. grilled, **Mexican cuisine, Moroccan cuisine**, mint, **Nuts**, **Onions**, oregano, papaya, passion fruit, paprika, parsley, peanuts, pork, poultry, quinoa, rum, salt, **Sauces**, sesame oil, **Seafood esp. shellf sh,** sugar, sweet potatoes, tequila, **Thai cuisine**, tomatoes, vanilla, vinegar, vodka, yogurt

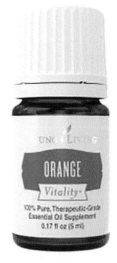

Orange (Tangerine)

Taste: sweet, citrusy

Temperature: warm

Intensity: mild - moderate

Timing: Add at the end of cooking process unless using in baked goods

Purpose: Orange oil adds a great burst of citrusy flavor to a dish without the acidity.

Pairs with:

Apples, apricots, anchovies, arugula, asparagus, avocado, bananas, basil, bay leaf, black pepper, beef, beets, beer esp. Blue Moon, **Berries**, bok choy, brussel sprouts, brandy, buttermilk, caramel, cardamom, carrots, cayenne, celery, ceviche, **Cheese esp. Firm goat**, cherries, chervil, chestnuts, chickpeas, chicken, chili peppers, chives, chocolate, cilantro, **Citrus fruit**, cinnamon, cloves, coconut, coffee, **Cognac**, crab, cranberries, cream, creme fraiche, cumin, custard, dates, desserts, duck esp. Duck a l'orange, eggplant, endive, escarole, fennel, figs, fish, game, garlic, ginger, grapefruit, grapes, green beans, guava, hazelnuts, juniper berries, kiwi, kumquats, lamb, leeks, lemon, lemongrass, lemon verbena, lettuce, lime, lychees, mango, melon, mint, nectarines, **Nuts**, oats, olives, olive oil, **Onions**, oregano, papaya, paprika, parsley, passion fruit, parsnips, peaches, pears, persimmons, pineapple, pistachios, plums, pomegranates, poppy seeds, pork, poultry, prunes, pumpkin,. quince, quinoa, raisins, rhubarb, rice, rosemary, rum, rutabaga, saffron, salad greens, salt, **Sauces esp. glazes**, sesame oil, **Seafood esp. scallops,** shallots, sherry, strawberries, squash (winter), swiss chard, sugar, thyme, tomatoes, vanilla, vinegar, vodka, walnuts, watercress, **Wine esp. port**, yogurt

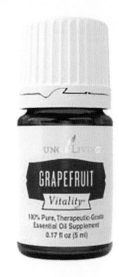

Grapefruit

Taste: bitter, citrusy

Temperature: warm

Intensity: strong

Timing: Add at the end of cooking process unless using in baked goods

Purpose: Grapefruit oil adds a bitter punch of citrusy flavor to dishes without the acidity.

Pairs with:

Arugula, asparagus, avocado, bananas, basil, beets, beer, caramel, cardamom, carrots, cayenne, celery, ceviche, chamgne, chervil, chestnuts, chickpeas, chicken, chili peppers, chives, cilantro, **Citrus fruit**, coconut, crab, cranberries, creme fraiche, desserts, fennel, **Fish**, ginger, guava, hazelnuts, honey, kiwi, kumquats, leeks, lemon, lemongrass, lemon verbena, lettuce, lime, melon, mint, nectarines, **Nuts**, olive oil, **Onions**, papaya, paprika, parsley, passion fruit, pineapple, pistachios, pomegranates, poppy seeds, port, poultry, rosemary, rum, salad greens, **Seafood esp. scallops,** seaweed, shallots, sorbet, spearmint, squash, strawberries, , sugar, tarragon, thyme, tomatoes, vanilla, vinegar, vinaigrette, vodka, walnuts, watercress, **Wine esp. sparkling**, yogurt

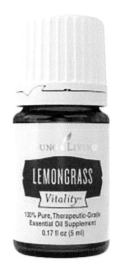

Lemon Grass

Taste: pungent, citrusy, herbaceous, floral

Temperature: hot

Intensity: moderate

Timing: Add in the beginning of cooking process

Purpose: Lemongrass is a unique aromatic that adds a citrusy floral hint to dishes.

Pairs with:

Asian cuisine, asparagus, beef, black pepper, bok choy, broccoli, brussel sprouts, butter, carrots, cauliflower, chicken, chili peppers, chives, cilantro, cinnamon, **Citrus fruit**, coconut, coconut milk, coriander, coriander, corn, crab, cumin, curries, dressings (salad), duck, edamame, eggplant, **Fish,** five-spice powder, garlic, ginger, green beans, honey, **Indonesian cuisine**, lamb, leeks, lemon, meats, mint, mushrooms, noodles, **Nuts**, okra, **Onions**, orange, parsley, parsnips, peanuts, **Peppers**, pineapple, pork, poultry, salt, **Sauces**, scallions, sesame oil, **Seafood esp. lobster,** shallots, soups, soy, soy sauce, snow peas, spinach, stocks, squash, stews, sweet potatoes, tea, **Thai cuisine**, turmeric, vanilla, veal, vegetables, **Vietnamese cuisine,** vinaigrettes, watercress

FLORAL OILS

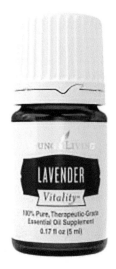

Lavender

Taste: semi-sweet, floral, citrusy

Temperature: mild

Intensity: strong

Timing: add in the beginning of cooking process especially when baked goods, or at the end as a garnish in either a sweet lipid like honey or infused oil

Purpose: Lavender adds complexity to a dish, as it is not a commonly used in traditional American fare. Without question, lavender adds a strong aromatic component to food.

Pairs with:

Apples, beef, **Berries**, **Cheese**, cherries, chicken, cream & ice cream, creme fraiche, currants, custards, desserts, duck, figs, fennel, **French cuisine**, fruits (cooked), garlic, ginger, honey, lamb, lemon (lemonade), marjoram, milk, mint, **Onions**, orange, oregano, parsley, peaches, plums, pork, poultry, potatoes, **Provencal cuisine**, quail, rabbit, rhubarb, rice, rosemary, sage, salt, savory, strawberries, sugar, tea, thyme, vanilla, vinegar esp. balsamic, walnuts

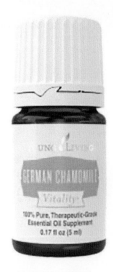

German Chamomile

Taste: slightly-sweet, floral

Temperature: mild

Intensity: mild - moderate

Timing: add at the beginning of the cooking process

Purpose: Chamomile comes in many varieties and the Vitality line has offered both Roman and German based on availability of it's whole plant form. All varieties exhibit a subtle apple-like flavor with floral scents. Chamomile adds an element of complexity to a dish

Pairs with:

Asian cuisine, apples, beverages esp. Hot tea, chicken, desserts, honey, lemon, **Meats esp. white meat**, rice, tea, veal

The Young Living Vitality Food Pairing Bible

GREEN HERB OILS

Basil

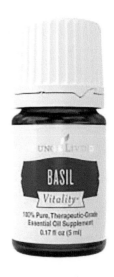

Taste: semi-floral, mildly herbaceous, light undertones of liquorice

Temperature: warm

Intensity: moderate

Timing: add towards the end of the cooking process

Purpose: Basil is used as an aromatic to compliment other flavors. It's usually dominated by other spices but works extremely well with the items below.

Pairs with:

Apples, apricots, **Asian cuisine**, asparagus, barley, bay leaf, beans, bean curd, beef, beets, **Berries**, black pepper, bok choy, broccoli, brussel sprouts, butter, capers, carrots, cayenne, cauliflower, **Cheese esp. Mozzarella, parmesan, feta**, chicken, chickpeas, chili peppers, chives, chocolate, cilantro, cinnamon, **Citrus fruit**, cinnamon, coconut, coconut milk, coriander, corn, crab, cranberries, cream & **Milk: cow, almond, soy, cashew, coconut**, creme fraiche, cucumber, cumin, custard, dates, dressing (salad), duck, edamame, **Eggs,** eggplant, endive, fennel, **Fish,** five-spice powder, **French cuisine**, garlic, ginger, green beans, hazelnuts, honey, **Italian cuisine**, kohlrabi, lamb, leeks, lemon, lemongrass, lettuce, lime, liver, marjoram, meats, **Mediterranean cuisine,** mint, mushrooms, mustard, nectarines, **Nuts**, okra, olives, olive oil, **Onions**, orange, oregano, parsley, parsnips, peaches, peanuts, pears, **Peppers**, pineapple, plums, pork, poultry, prunes, quince, quinoa, rosemary, salt, **Sauces**, scallions, sesame oil, **Seafood,** shallots, sherry, soups, soy, soy sauce, snow peas, pesto, spinach, stocks, squash, sugar, sweet potatoes, **Thai cuisine,** thyme, **Tomatoes,** vanilla, veal, vegetables, vinegar, **Vietnamese cuisine,** watercress, watermelon, wine,

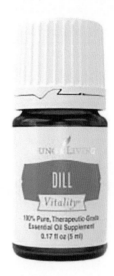

Dill

Taste: semi-sweet, herbaceous, pungent

Temperature: warm

Intensity: strong

Timing: add towards the end of the cooking process

Purpose: Dill adds a grassy freshness to foods. Even diluted in a carrier oil, a little goes a long way.

Pairs with:

Anchovies, artichokes, asparagus, avocado, basil, black pepper, beans, bread's, broccoli, butter, capers, carrots, cauliflower, celery, **Cheese esp. Goat varieties**, chervil, chestnuts, chicken, chili peppers, chives, corn, crab, cream & **Milk: cow, almond, soy, cashew, coconut**, creme fraiche, cumin, cucumbers, **Eggs**, eggplant, endive, **Fish,** garlic, **German cuisine, Greek cuisine**, green beans, horseradish, lemon, lettuce, **Mediterranean cuisine**, mint, mushrooms, mustard, **Nuts**, **Onions**, parsley, parsnips, peas, pickles, **Potatoes**, poultry, **Russian cuisine,** salads, salt, **Sauces, Seafood esp. shellfish**, sour cream, spinach, squash, thyme, tomatoes, veal, vegetables, yogurt and yogurt sauces

Sage

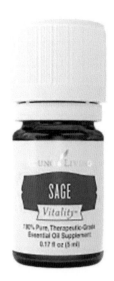

Taste: savory, herbaceous, umami

Temperature: warm

Intensity: moderate - strong

Timing: add at the beginning of the cooking process, or at the end if using as garnish (sage infused oil)

Purpose: Sage is an aromatic that imparts an extremely savory element to foods. It alone taste like thanksgiving. It's recommended to split the drop (using the formula) if adding directly into a recipe.

Pairs with:

Acorn squash, allspice, apples, asparagus, bacon, basil, bay leaf, black pepper, **Beef, Berries, Beans fresh and dried,** brussel sprouts, butter, buttermilk, butternut squash, cabbage, capers, caramel, caraway, carrots, cardamom, cauliflower, celery, **Cheese esp. Brie, Gruyere,** chestnuts, **Chicken**, chives, **Citrus fruit**, cinnamon, corn, cranberries, cream & **Milk: cow, almond, soy, cashew, coconut**, dates, duck, eggs, eggplant, endive, fennel, figs, **Fish, French cuisine,** garlic, ginger, **Greek cuisine**, honey, lamb, lemon, **Liver esp. Foie gras**, marjoram, **Meats, Mediterranean cuisine,** mint, mushrooms, mustard, **Nuts**, olive oil, **Onions**, orange, oregano, paprika, parsley, parsnips, pasta, peaches, pears, peas, **Pork, Poultry,** pumpkin,, rosemary, rutabaga, salt, **Sausages, Seafood esp. shellfish,** shallots, sherry, soups, **Spanish cuisine**, stews, **stuffing**, sugar, thyme, tomatoes, turkey, veal, vegetables, walnuts, **Wine esp. white**

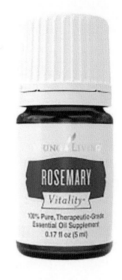

Rosemary

Taste: pungent, piney, woodsy

Temperature: warm

Intensity: moderate - strong

Timing: add at the beginning of the cooking process

Purpose: Rosemary adds an extreme aromatic component to dishes that imparts a deep rustic flavor on the pallete. Rosemary does not play nice with others and can easily dominate a dish. It's recommended to split the drop (using the formula) if adding directly into a recipe or start with a teaspoon of infused rosemary oil in your recipe instead of using drops all together.

Pairs with:

Acorn squash, allspice, anchovies, apples, asparagus, bacon, basil, bay leaf, black pepper, **Beef, Berries, Beans fresh and dried, Breads esp. focaccia** , brussel sprouts, butter, buttermilk, butternut squash, cabbage, capers, carrots, cauliflower, celery, **Cheese esp. Brie, Gruyere,** chestnuts, **Chicken**, chives, **Citrus fruit**, cranberries, cream & **Milk: cow, almond, soy, cashew,** dates, duck, eggs, eggplant, endive, fennel, figs, **Fish**, **French cuisine**, fruit, **Game esp. venison**, garlic, grapefruit, honey, lamb, lavender, lemon, lentils, lime,**Liver esp. calf's**, marjoram, marinades, **Meats grilled, roasted, esp. sous vide**, **Mediterranean cuisine**, mint, mushrooms, mustard, **Nuts**, octopus, olive oil, **Onions**, orange, oregano, pancetta, parsley, parsnips, pasta, **Pastries**, pears, peas, pizza, **Pork**, potatoes, **Poultry**, pumpkin, radicchio, risotto, sage, salt, **Seafood esp. Salmon**, sardines, sauces, savory, shallots, sherry, shrimp, soups, spinach, speck, stews, strawberries, sweet potatoes, thyme, tomatoes, turkey, veal, vegetables, vinegar, balsamic, walnuts, **Wine esp. white**, zucchini

Marjoram

Taste: semi-sweet, herbaceous

Temperature: warm

Intensity: moderate

Timing: add towards the end of cooking process

Purpose: Marjoram adds a light herbaceous element to foods that is complimentary versus being overpowering. It's often regarded as a light oregano.

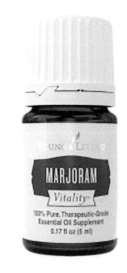

Pairs with:

Apples, anchovies, artichokes, arugula, asparagus, basil, bay leaf, black pepper, beef, beets, Beans esp.dry, bouquet garni (key ingredient), brussel sprouts, buckwheat, butter, buttermilk, carrots, cayenne, cauliflower, celery, **Cheese: parmesan, mascarpone**, chickpeas, chicken, chili peppers, chives, chowders, clams, corn, crab, cream, creme fraiche, cucumber, dressings esp. vinaigrette, duck, eggs, eggplant, escarole, figs, **Fish, French cuisine**, fines herbes (key ingredient), garlic, ginger **Greek cuisine**, green beans, Italian cuisine, lamb, **lemon,** lima beans, meats, **Mediterranean cuisine**, mint, **Moroccan cuisine**, mushrooms, mustard, **Nuts**, olives, olive oil, **Onions**, oregano, parsley, parsnips, pasta, peas, plums, pork, potatoes, poultry, risotto, rosemary, rutabaga, sage, salt, salad greens, **Sauces**, savory dishes, **Seafood esp. Clams, halibut,** shallots, sherry, spinach, soups, stews, squash, swiss chard, thyme, tomatoes, vegetables esp. Summer, vinegar, vodka, walnuts, watercress, **Wine**, zucchini

Oregano

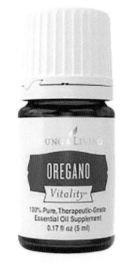

Taste: pungent, herbaceous, spicy

Temperature: hot

Intensity: strong

Timing: Add in the beginnning of the cooking process

Purpose: Oregano adds an intense herbaceous flavor to recipes. It too, has a rustic component that has the potential to take over a dish. It's recommended to split the drop (using the formula) if adding directly into a recipe. Oregano oil makes a great infused oil that can be added at the end of the cooking process if you desire deeper flavor. The cooking process rounds out oregano oils harsh flavor and heat.

Pairs with:

Anchovies, artichokes, arugula, asparagus, basil, bay leaf, black pepper, beef, beets, bell peppers, **Beans esp.dry**, broccoli, broccoli rabe, broths, butter, capers, carrots, **Cheese parmesan, feta**, chickpeas, chicken, chili peppers, chimichurri, chives, corn, creme fraiche, cucumbers, dressings, duck, eggs, eggplant, escarole, **Fish, French cuisine**, garlic, **Greek cuisine**, green beans, grilled dishes, **Italian cuisine**, lamb, leeks, **Lemon,** lima beans, **Meats**, meatballs, **Mediterranean cuisine**, mint, mole sauces, mushrooms, mussels, mustard, **Nuts**, olives, olive oil, **Onions**, paprika, parsley, parsnips, **Pasta**, pizza, peas, polenta, pork, potatoes, poultry, radicchio, risotto, rosemary, rutabaga, sage, salt, salads, salad greens, **Sauces**, savory dishes, **Seafood esp. swordfish,** s hallots, shrimp, sherry, spinach, soups, **Spanish cuisine**, squash, stews, stuffing, swiss chard, thyme, **Tomatoes esp. Tomato sauces**, veal, vegetables esp. Summer, vinaigrettes, vinegar, walnuts, watercress, **Wine**, zucchini

Peppermint

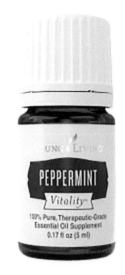

Taste: sweet, cooling, pungent

Temperature: warm

Intensity: strong

Timing: Add at the beginning of the cooking process (if using in baked goods add directly to the fat called for in the recipe

Purpose: Peppermint adds an extreme menthol like flavor that creates a chilling sensation in dishes. It's high concetration of menthol limits its application in the kitchen to mostly sweet foods.

Pairs with:

Apples, **Berries**, **Beverages esp. Hot tea & hot chocolate**, brownies, cakes, candies, cream & ice cream, chocolate, coffee, cottage cheese, custards, desserts, honey, lamb, lemon, milk, mint, oatmeal, **Pastries,** strawberries, sugar, teas, truffles, waffles, whipped cream, white chocolate

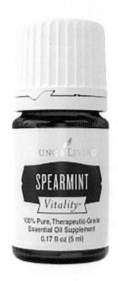

Spearmint

Taste: sweet, mild-cooling, herbaceous

Temperature: warm

Intensity: moderate

Timing: Add at the beginning of the cooking process

Purpose: Spearmint adds a subtle refreshing herbaceous essence to foods that isn't overpowering. Spearmint blends well with other ingredients and can be used in countless ways to mimic foods from cultures around the globe.

Pairs with:

Apples, beef, beets, **Berries**, **Beverages esp. Hot tea & hot chocolate**, brownies, bulgar, butter, cakes, candies, cantaloupe, cream & ice cream, cheese esp. Feta, chicken esp. grilled, chocolate, coffee, cottage, couscous, custards, cucumbers, duck, desserts, garlic, **Greek cuisine**, gyros, harissa, honey, hummus, kebabs, lamb, leeks, lemon, lentils esp. Lentil salad, iced tea, **Meats**, **Mediterranean cuisine,** melon, meyer lemon, milk, mint, mojito, oatmeal, olive oil, olives, onions, oregano, **Pastries, Portuguese cuisine esp. Rice**, pea, pork, raisins, savory dishes, spanakopita, spinach, snow peas, strawberries, sugar, tabbouleh, tomatoes & tomato sauces, teas, truffles, **Turkish cuisine**, waffles, watermelon, yogurt, zucchini

Tarragon

Flavor: bitter-sweet, licorice, herbaceous

Temperature: warm

Intensity: moderate - strong

Timing: add in the beggining of cooking process, or at the end if using as garnish (tarragon infused oil)

Purpose: Tarragon adds a semi sweet herbaceous flavor to foods. It's tends to compliment other ingredients by extending the flavor sensations for longer durations.

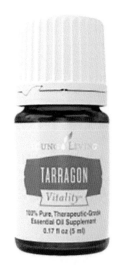

Pairs with:

Aioli, apples, apricots, anchovies, asparagus, avocado, balsamic, basil, bay leaf, black pepper, beef, beets, Bearnaise (key ingredient), brussel sprouts, brandy, broccoli, buttermilk, capers, carrots, cayenne, celery, **Cheese esp. Brie, blue cheese**, chervil, chestnuts, chickpeas, chicken, chili peppers, chives, chocolate, cilantro, **Citrus fruit**, cinnamon, cloves, coconut, coffee, **Cognac**, collard greens, corn, crab, cranberries, cream, creme fraiche, cumin, custard, dates, desserts, dill, eggs, eggplant, endive, escarole, fennel, fennel seeds, fines herbes (key ingredient), fish, **French cuisine**, frisee, game esp. birds, garlic, grapes, grapefruit, green beans, guava, hazelnuts, juniper berries, kale, kiwi, kumquats, lamb, leeks, lemon, lemongrass, lemon verbena, lettuce, lime, lobster, mango, marjoram, **Meats,** melon, mint, mushrooms, mustard, nectarines, **Nuts**, oats esp. Steel cut, olives, olive oil, **Onions**, orange, papaya, paprika, parsley, parsnips, peaches, pears, peas, Pernod (Anise liqueur), pistachios, pomegranates, pork, potatoes, **Poultry esp. turkey**, quinoa, radishes, raisins, rice, salad greens, salt, **Sauces, Seafood esp. Halibut, shellfish,** shallots, sherry, soups, sorrel, soy sauce, spinach, strawberries, squash (summer), tomatoes, veal, vegetables, vinaigrette, vinegar, **Wine, red**, zucchini

Thyme

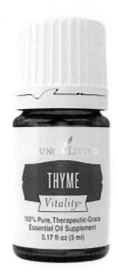

Taste: pungent, piney, woodsy

Temperature: warm

Intensity: strong

Timing: add in the beginning of cooking process (It also makes for a great infused oil)

Purpose: Although thyme is considered a strong aromatic, it imparts a mild woodsy flavor to a dishes. It blends extremely well with other green herbs to create extremely balanced flavors. Beware, it can easily take over a dish with 1 drop to many.

Pairs with:

Allspice, apples, apricots, asparagus, bacon, barley, bay leaf, beans, beef, beets, **Berries**, black pepper, bouquet garni (key ingredient), braised dishes, broccoli, brussel sprouts, butter, cabbage, capers, carrots, cayenne, cauliflower, **Cheese esp. Mozzarella, parmesan, feta**, chicken, chickpeas, chili peppers, chives, chocolate, chowders, cilantro, cinnamon, **Citrus fruit**, cinnamon, cloves, coriander, corn, crab, cranberries, curries, cream, creme fraiche, cumin, dates, dill, duck, **Eggs,** eggplant, endive, fennel, **Fish, French cuisine**, fruits, dried, garlic, **Greek cuisine,** green beans, gumbos, herbes de Provence, hazelnuts, honey, **Italian cuisine, Jamaican cuisine**, jambalaya, jerk paste, seasoning, kohlrabi, lamb, lavender, leeks, legumes, lemon, lime, liver, marinades, marjoram, **Meats esp. Oven roasted, Mediterranean cuisine, Middle Eastern cuisine**, mint, mole sauce, mushrooms, mustard, **Nuts**, nutmeg, olives, olive oil, **Onions**, orange, oregano, paprika, parsley, parsnips, pasta, pate, peaches, peanuts, pears, **Peppers**, pineapple, pizza, plums, pork, poultry, quinoa, rice, rosemary, sage, salt, **Sauces esp. Beurre, demi-glace**, savory, scallops, **Seafood,** shallots, sherry, soups, soy sauce, snow peas, spinach, stews, stocks, stuffings, squash, tarragon, tomatoes, veal, vegetables, vinaigrettes, vinegar, **Wine esp. Wine sauces**, zucchin

Mountain Savory

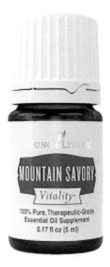

Taste: herbaceous, spicy-peppery, woosy

Temperature: warm

Intensity: moderate - strong

Timing: add at the beginning of the cooking process

Purpose: As the name suggest savory adds a deep woodsy element to a dish with a little kick. It's an extremely strong aromatic

Pairs with:

Acorn squash, basil, bay leaf, black pepper, **Beef**, beets, bell peppers, bouquet garni, **Beans fresh and dried**, brussel sprouts, butternut squash, cabbage, carrots, celery, chestnuts, **Chicken**, chicken livers, chives, cumin, cranberries, duck, eggs, eggplant, fennel, figs, **Fish**, fines herbes, garlic, herbes de Provence (key ingredient), lamb, lavender, leeks, legumes, lemon, lentils, **Meats, esp. grilled, roasted, Mediterranean cuisine**, mint, mushrooms, nutmeg, olives, olive oil, **Onions**, oregano, pancetta, parsley, parsnips, peas, polenta, **Pork**, potatoes, **Poultry**, pumpkin, rice, risotto, root vegetables, rosemary, sage, salt, sauces, shallots, sherry, soups, spinach, stews, sweet potatoes, tarragon, thyme, tomatoes, veal, vegetables, vinegar, **Wine esp. red**, zucchini

KITCHEN CLASSICS OILS

Black Pepper

Taste: pungent, spicy-hot, earthy

Temperature: warm

Intensity: moderate - strong

Timing: add at the beginning of the cooking process, or as a garnish (black pepper infused oil)

Purpose: Black pepper is one of the most revered spices around the world. It adds a subtle element of heat and depth of flavor to almost any dish.

Pairs with:

Apricots, asparagus, bay leaf, beans, beef, beets, **Berries**, bok choy, broccoli, brussel sprouts, butter, capers, carrots, cauliflower, **Cheese**, chicken, chick peas, chili peppers, chives, coconut milk, coriander, corn, creme fraiche, cucumber, cumin, dressing (salad), duck, edamame, **Eggs,** garlic, ginger, kale, lamb, lemon, lime, **Meats esp. steak**, mushrooms, mustard, **Nuts**, olives, olive oil, **Onions**, orange, oregano, parsley, parsnips, peaches, peanuts, pears, **Peppers**, pineapple, pork, poultry, pumpkin, rosemary, salads, salt, **Sauces, Seafood,** shallots, sherry, soups, soy, soy sauce, snow peas, spinach, stocks, squash, sugar, sweet potatoes, thyme, tomatoes, veal, vegetables, vinegar, watercress, watermelon, wine,

Celery Seed

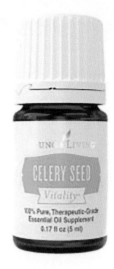

Taste: slightly sweet, grassy, celery

Temperature: mild

Intensity: moderate

Timing: add at the beginning of the cooking process

Purpose: Celery seed is pungent aromatic that adds celery-like flavor to foods.

Pairs with:

Allspice, aioli, apples, bay leaf, beef, breads, **Cajun/Creole cuisine**, celery root, cheese, chervil, carrots, cauliflower, chicken, coriander, dill, eggplant, eggs, fennel seeds, garlic, **German cuisine**, ginger, **Indian cuisine**, lamb, legumes, lemon, lime, **Meats**, mushrooms, mustard, onions, paprika, peas, parsnips, **Pastries**, peaches, pears, **Peppers**, potatoes, poultry, **Russian cuisine**, salads, **Sauces**, shallots, shellfish, stews, stocks, thyme, tomatoes, vegetables, Worcestershire sauce

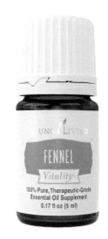

Fennel

Taste: semisweet, strong liquorice

Temperature: mild

Intensity: mild - moderate

Timing: add at the beginning of the cooking process

Purpose: Fennel imparts a moderate floral element to dishes with a strong anise flavor. It adds layers of flavor to traditional foods.

Pairs with:

Anise, apples, arugula, asparagus, bacon, basil, bay leaf, black pepper, beef, beets, butter, carrots, capers, **Cheese esp. parmesan**, chicken, chili peppers, chives, crab, cranberries, cream, creme fraiche, dill, duck, eggplant, endive, escarole, figs, frisee, garlic, ginger, greens (salad), green beans, honey, **Italian cuisine**, lamb, leeks, lemon, lime, lettuce, lobster, **Mediterranean cuisine**, mint, mussels, nutmeg, olives, olive oil, **Onions**, orange, oregano, pancetta, papaya, paprika, parsley, parsnips, pasta, peaches, pears, **Pernod liquor**, pork, poultry, potatoes, prosciutto, rosemary, salt, **Sauces**, scallions, **Seafood esp. shellfish,** shallots, sherry, sour cream, spinach, squash, swiss chard, sugar, tarragon, thyme, tomatoes, vinaigrettes, vinegar, walnuts, watercress, **Wine**, yogurt

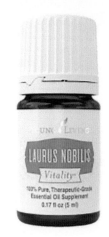

Laurus Nobilis (Bay Leaf)

Taste: pungent, piney,

Temperature: hot

Intensity: moderate - strong

Timing: Add in the beginning of cooking process

Purpose: Bay leaf, by its very nature, plays second fiddle to other, more prominent flavors. However, it's often that something that's missing when it's not in a dish. Overall this potent aromatic tends to balance other spices and ingredients by imparting a pleasant eucalyptus-like flavor to dishes.

Pairs with:

Allspice, apples, barley, beans, basil, black pepper, braised recipes, broth, cashews, cauliflower, celery, chestnuts, chicken, chives, corn, cream, duck, dumplings (American), figs, fish, forcemeat, **French cuisine**, garlic, grains, juniper berries, hazelnuts, lamb, **Legumes esp. lentils, white beans**, leeks, lemon, marinades, marjoram, **Meats esp. crockpot**, **Mediterranean cuisine**, mole sauce, olive oil, olives, **Onions**, parsley, pears, polenta, pork, pot roast, potatoes, **Poultry**, pumpkin, quail, quinoa, **Rice esp. pilaf**, rosemary, sage, salt, **Sauces**, **Seafood**, soups, spinach, squash, stews, stocks, thyme, tomatoes, turkey, vanilla, veal, venison, vinegar, walnuts, **Wine`**

The Young Living Vitality Food Pairing Bible

SWEET SPICE OILS

Ginger

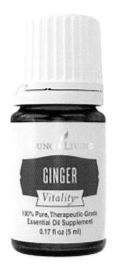

Taste: semi-bitter, pungent, spicy

Temperature: warm (spicy)

Intensity: strong

Timing: add in the beggining of cooking process, or at the end if using as garnish (ginger infused oil)

Purpose: Ginger imparts a spicy umami flavor in foods. It's also commonly revered to aid digestive support.

Pairs with:

Allspice, anise, apples, apricots, **Asian cuisine**, asparagus, bananas, barley, basil, bay leaf, beans, bean curd, beef, beets, black pepper, bok choy, broccoli, brussel sprouts, buckwheat, butter, caramel, cardamom, carrots, cayenne, cauliflower, celery, **Cheese esp. brie**, chickpeas, chicken, chili peppers, chives, chocolate, cilantro, cinnamon, **Citrus fruit**, cider, cinnamon, coconut, coriander, coffee, corn, crab, cranberries, cream & **Milk: cow, almond, soy, cashew, coconut**, creme fraiche, cumin, custard, dates, desserts, dressing (salad), duck, edamame, eggplant, endive, figs, five-spice powder, garlic, grapefruit, green beans, guava, hazelnuts, honey, **Indian cuisine, Indonesian cusine, Japanese cuisine,** kaffir lime leaves, kale, **Korean cuisine**, kohlrabi, lamb, lavender, leeks, lemon, lemongrass, lemon verbena, lettuce, lime, lychees, mangoes, **Middle Eastern cuisine**, mint, molasses, **Moroccan cuisine**, mushrooms, noodles, **North African cuisine**, **Nuts**, nutmeg, oats, okra, olives, olive oil, **Onions**, orange, papaya, parsley, parsnips, passion fruit, peaches, peanuts, pears, **Peppers**, persimmons, pineapple, plums, pork, poultry, prunes, pumpkin, quince, quinoa, raisins, rhubarb, rice, rum, saffron, salt, **Sauces**, scallions, sesame oil, **Seafood,** shallots, sherry, soups, soy, soy sauce, snow peas, spinach, star anise, strawberries, stocks, squash, sugar, sushi, sweet potatoes, tamarind, tarragon, tea, **Thai cuisine,** tomatoes, turmeric, vanilla, vegetables, vinegar, **Vietnamese cuisine, Vinegar esp. Rice wine**, watercress, wasabi, wine, yogurt, yuzu

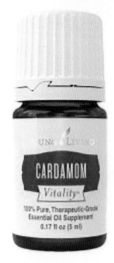

Cardamom

Taste: nutty, citrusy, bitter

Temperature: warm

Intensity: moderate - strong

Timing: add at the beginning of the cooking process

Purpose: Cardamom adds a deliteful bitterness to foods and is often associted with the idea of balancing a dish.

Pairs with:

Anise, apples, apricots, bananas, beef, beets, beverages esp. hot, bok choy, broccoli, brussel sprouts, butter, caraway, carrots, cauliflower, chicken, chick peas, chili peppers, chocolate, cinnamon, coconut milk, coriander, corn, creme anglaise, cumin, curry, custards, dates, desserts, duck, garam masala, garlic, ginger, honey, **Indian cuisine**, lamb, legumes, lemon, lime, **Meats esp. red**, **Nuts**, orange, paprika, parsnips, **Pastries**, peaches,pears, **Peppers**, pineapple, pork, poultry, pumpkin, saffron, **Sauces**, shallots, soups, spinach, stocks, squash, sugar, sweet potatoes, tea, tomatoes, vegetables, walnuts, wine yogurt

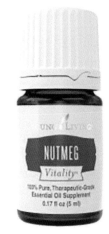

Nutmeg

Taste: sweet, nutty, spicy

Temperature: warm

Intensity: strong

Timing: add at the beginning of the cooking process

Purpose: Nutmeg is an extremely versatile aromatic that leans in the direction of how its used. It blends well with other sweet spices, but can be powerful on its own to add extraordinary depth of flavor to dishes.

Pairs with:

Allspice, anise, apples, apricots, beef, **Berries**, beverages esp. hot, broccoli, butter, cabbage, caramel, cardamom, **Caribbean cuisine**, carrots, cauliflower, cheese esp. Ricotta (mac & cheese), chicken, chili peppers, chili powder, chives, **Chinese cuisine**, chocolate, chowders (corn), cinnamon, cloves, coconut, compotes, coriander, coffee, cream, cumin, curries, custard, dates, desserts, eggs, eggnog, eggplant, escarole, figs, five-spice powder, French toast, **French cuisine**, fruits, garam masala, **German cuisine**, ginger, hazelnuts, honey, **Indian cuisine, Italian cuisine, Jerk seasoning**, lamb, lemon, mace, malt, **Meats**, mushrooms, **Nuts**, oats, okra, **Onions**, orange, pancakes, parsnips, **Pastries esp. cookies, cakes**, pate, peaches, peanuts, pears, pecans, plums, pork, poultry, pumpkin, quail, quinoa, raisins, rice, **Sauces esp. White, cream**, sausages, **Scandinavian cuisine**, spinach, **Seafood esp. Bisque**, soups, sour cream, star anise, stocks, squash, sugar, sweet potatoes, swiss chard, thyme, tarragon, vanilla, wine, yogurt

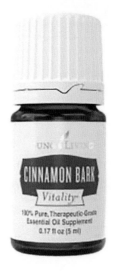

Cinnamon Bark

Taste: semi-bitter, sweet, woodsy, spicy

Temperature: hot

Intensity: strong

Timing: add at the beginning of the cooking process

Purpose: Cinnamon adds a spicy warming component to dishes. It's an extremely pungent aromatic with a distinct flavor.

Pairs with:

Allspice, anise, apples esp. cider , apricots, bananas, beef, bell peppers, **Berries**, beverages, esp. hot, tea, butter, caramel, cardamom, carrots, cherries, chicken, chili peppers, chili powder, chives, chocolate, coconut, compotes, coriander, coffee, cloves, cookies, cranberries, cream & **Milk: cow, almond, soy, cashew, coconut**, cumin, curries, custard, dates, desserts, eggplant, fennel, figs, five-spice powder (key ingredient), French toast, fruits, garam masala, garlic, ginger, hazelnuts, honey, **Indian cuisine, Indonesian cuisine,** kohlrabi, lamb, lemon, mace, malt, **Meats esp. Red**, **Mexican cuisine**, molasses, **Moroccan cuisine**, nutmeg, oats, okra, **Onions**, orange, pancakes, **Pastries**, parsnips, peaches, peanuts, pears, pecans, **Peppers**, plums, pork, poultry, prunes, pumpkin, quail, quinoa, raisins, rhubarb, rice, rum, saffron, salt, **Sauces**, soups, star anise, stocks, squash, sugar, sweet potatoes, tamarind, tarragon, tea, tomatoes, turmeric, vanilla, vegetables, waffles, wine, yogurt, zucchini

Coriander

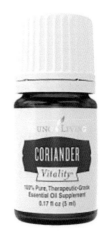

Taste: citrusy, earthy, semi-sweet

Temperature: cool

Intensity: mild - moderate

Timing: add at the beginning of the cooking process

Purpose: Coriander is a flavor enhancer that blends well with other spices. It imparts a desirable citrusy earthiness to dishes with a hint of spice.

Pairs with:

Allspice, anise, apples, bacon, beef, bell peppers, caramel, cardamom, carrots, chicken, chili peppers, chili powder, chocolate, cilantro, cinnamon, **Citrus,** coconut, coconut milk, compotes, cloves, cumin, curries, desserts, fennel, fennel seeds, figs, fish, garam masala, garlic, ginger, grapefruit, ham, harissa, honey, lamb, **Latin American cuisine**, lemongrass, lentils, mace, malt, **Meats**, **Mediterranean cuisine, Mexican cuisine**, **Middle Eastern cuisine**, mint, **Moroccan cuisine**, nutmeg, oats, **Onions**, orange, **Pastries**, pears, pecans, **Peppers**, plums, pork, potatoes, poultry, pumpkin, quail, quince, quinoa, raisins, rhubarb, rice, rum, saffron, salt, sesame seeds, star anise, stews, stocks, squash, sugar, sweet potatoes, tomatoes, turmeric, vanilla, vegetables, waffles, wine, yogurt, zucchini

CULINARY MASTER BLENDS

All master blends based on a mixture of 1 cup of lipid (light olive oil recommended)

- Basil (4 drops) + Oregano (1 drop)
- Fennel (2 drops) + Basil (2 drops) + Spearmint (1 drop)
- Lemon (3 drops) + Black Pepper (2 drops)
- Orange (4 drops) + Rosemary (1 drop)
- Lemon (4 drops) + Rosemary (1 drop)
- Lemon (4 drops) + Oregano (1 drop)
- Lemon (3 drops) + Marjoram (1 drop)
- Lemon (3 drops) + Mountain Savory (2 drops)
- Cinnamon Bark (2 drops) + Cardamom (2 drops)
- Cinnamon Bark (1 drops) + Nutmeg (1 drop) + Cloves (1 drop) + Cardamom (1 drop) + Ginger (1 drop)
- Cinnamon Bark (1 drops) + Cardamom (1 drop) + Cloves (1 drop) + Coriander (1 drop)
- Dill (2 drops) + Lime (3 drops)
- Dill (2 drops) + Lemon (3 drops)
- Basil (2 drops) + Rosemary (1 drop) + Thyme (1drop) + Oregano (1drop)
- Savory (1 drop) + Marjoram (1 drop) + Lavender (1 drop) + Rosemary (1 drop) + Thyme (1 drop)
- Sage (1 drop) + Thyme (1 drop) + Marjoram (1 drop) + Rosemary (1 drop) + Celery Seed (1 drop) + Black Pepper (1 drop)
- Oregano (1 drop) + Basil (1 drop) + Thyme (1 drop) + Savory (1 drop) + Coriander (1 drop) + Black Pepper (1 drop)
- Ginger (3 drops) + Lemon Grass (2 drops)
- Ginger (3 drops) + Cloves (2 drops)
- Ginger (1 drops) + Lemon (3 drops) + Spearmint (1 drop)
- Fennel (1 drop) + Lemon (3 drops) + Spearmint (1 drop)
- Fennel (1 drop) + Orange (3 drops) + Tarragon (1 drop)
- Orange (3 drops) + Tarragon (2 drops)
- Grapefruit (3 drops) + Spearmint (2 drops)
- Grapefruit (3 drops) + Fennel (2 drops)
- Spearmint (3 drops) + Dill (1 drop) + Coriander (1 drop)
- Nutmeg (3 drops) + Cloves (2 drops)
- Sage (2 drops) + Marjoram (drops) + Thyme (1 drop)
- Mountain Savory (3 drops) + Thyme (2 drops)

Printed in Germany
by Amazon Distribution
GmbH, Leipzig

31258230R00029